AUTOIMMUNE PROTOCOL DISEASE DIET COOKBOOK

Healing Recipes For Managing Inflammation, Boosting Immunity, And Restoring Gut Health With Paleo And Gluten-Free Meals

DR ELIAN GRIFFIN

DISCLAIMER

The nutritional recommendations and recipes in this book are meant solely for informative reasons. They are not meant to replace the counsel, diagnosis, or care of a qualified medical expert. If you have any doubts about a medical condition or dietary requirements, you should always see your physician or another trained healthcare expert.

All reasonable efforts have been taken by the author and publisher to ensure that the information contained in this book is correct as of the date of publication. Recommendations may alter, though, as medical knowledge is always changing. When using any of the recipes or instructions found here, the user assumes all liability and assumes no risk, whether personal or otherwise. People who have certain dietary requirements or medical issues should speak with a healthcare provider for personalized guidance. The given recipes are only ideas; you may need to adjust them to suit your own nutritional needs, tastes, and tolerances.

When you use this book, you agree to release the publisher, the author, and their representatives from any liability for any claims, damages, liabilities, costs, or expenditures resulting from your use of the book.

TABLE OF CONTENTS

ABOUT THE BOOK

"Autoimmune Protocol Disease Diet Cookbook" is a vital resource for anyone looking to control autoimmune conditions with dietary modifications. Autoimmune diseases, which impact millions of people globally and cause a variety of crippling symptoms that greatly affect day-to-day living, are defined in this book along with examples of common symptoms like inflammation, fatigue, and chronic pain.

It also emphasizes the critical role that diet plays in controlling these symptoms and presents the Autoimmune Protocol (AIP) Diet as a useful dietary approach.

With an emphasis on nutrient-dense foods, the book presents research supporting the effectiveness of the AIP diet in reducing autoimmune symptoms. Readers will gain a thorough understanding of how this diet can help manage their condition and improve their overall well-being. The book delves into the science behind the AIP diet, exploring its anti-inflammatory benefits and its positive impact on gut health and immune system modulation.

The AIP diet can be intimidating at first, but this book offers helpful advice on how to get started. It lists foods to include and avoid, offers meal-planning ideas, and recommends essential items for your shopping list. It also offers tips on how to set up your kitchen for the AIP journey. AIP diet transitions are thoroughly discussed, including the differences between gradual and immediate transitions, how to handle cravings and withdrawals, where to find resources and support, how to track your progress, and how to set realistic goals.

AIP diets require the avoidance of specific foods; the book explains common allergens, processed and refined foods, inflammatory foods, and hidden ingredients to look out for. It also teaches readers how to read and understand food labels so they can make educated decisions. Weekly meal planning tips, batch cooking and meal prep techniques, and AIP-friendly breakfast, lunch, and dinner recipes are all included in the book, making it simple to maintain a varied and enjoyable diet.

To ensure that readers have a plethora of delectable and compliant recipes to choose from, keeping their diet both satisfying and health-promoting, the cookbook section features a variety of AIP recipes, including breakfast options, lunch and dinner meals, snacks, desserts, smoothies, drinks, and special occasion meals. Snack and dessert ideas are also plentiful, with quick and easy snack ideas, healthy AIP desserts, portable snack options, and tips for making AIP treats, helping readers stay satisfied in between meals.

Eating out and traveling while following the AIP diet can be difficult, but this book offers helpful advice on how to locate AIP-friendly eateries, explain dietary requirements to others, pack meals and snacks for travel, and keep a healthy diet while on vacation. It also covers how to handle social gatherings where food is involved, so readers can follow their diet in a variety of situations.

Another important part of the AIP journey is managing cravings and emotional eating. The book offers healthy alternatives to common cravings, explains how to manage cravings and emotional eating, and discusses mindfulness, stress management, and creating a supportive environment to support dietary adherence.

Long-term success on the AIP diet depends on tracking progress and making necessary dietary adjustments. The book suggests journaling about food and symptoms, identifying and reintroducing foods, and modifying the diet in response to symptoms. It also stresses the value of collaborating with healthcare providers and acknowledging small victories.

A thorough FAQ section answers common questions about handling social situations, budget-friendly meals, dining out, supplements, and handling setbacks. This ensures that readers have all the information they need to successfully navigate the AIP diet and manage their autoimmune condition.

CHAPTER ONE

AUTOIMMUNE PROTOCOL DISEASE DIET INTRODUCTION

DEFINITION AND ILLUSTRATIONS

Autoimmune diseases are caused when the body's immune system attacks its tissues inadvertently, resulting in tissue damage and chronic inflammation. Common autoimmune diseases include lupus, multiple sclerosis, rheumatoid arthritis, and Hashimoto's thyroiditis. These conditions can affect the joints, skin, brain, and internal organs. It is important to understand autoimmune diseases because each person's symptoms vary, making diagnosis and treatment difficult.

Identification of the specific autoimmune condition helps to customize the treatment and management plan to the individual's needs. Autoimmune diseases are often diagnosed through a combination of symptoms, medical history, and laboratory tests that identify specific antibodies or markers in the blood.

For example, lupus can affect multiple organ systems, causing symptoms ranging from skin rashes to kidney problems.

Understanding the nature of autoimmune diseases and the available treatments is the first step toward effectively managing these chronic conditions. Living with an autoimmune disease often requires ongoing medical care and lifestyle adjustments.

Medications, such as immunosuppressants and anti-inflammatory drugs, are commonly prescribed to manage symptoms and prevent flare-ups. In addition to medical treatment, many patients benefit from complementary therapies like physical therapy, acupuncture, and stress management techniques.

TYPICAL SYMPTOMS

A person's quality of life can be greatly affected by common autoimmune disease symptoms, which can vary greatly depending on the particular condition.

Common symptoms of autoimmune diseases include fatigue, joint pain, skin rashes, and digestive problems. Fatigue is a common symptom across many autoimmune diseases and can interfere with daily activities and overall productivity.

Skin rashes and lesions are also common, especially in diseases like lupus and psoriasis. These skin issues can be both physically uncomfortable and emotionally distressing, affecting a person's self-esteem and social interactions. Joint pain and swelling are hallmark symptoms of autoimmune conditions like rheumatoid arthritis and lupus. This pain can range from mild discomfort to debilitating, making movement and daily tasks challenging.

An individual's health may be further complicated by digestive issues, such as bloating, diarrhea, and abdominal pain, which are commonly observed in autoimmune conditions such as Crohn's disease and celiac disease. Understanding these common symptoms is essential for early diagnosis and efficient management of autoimmune diseases, enabling individuals to seek appropriate medical care and support.

EFFECTS ON DAY-TO-DAY LIVING

Autoimmune diseases can have a significant impact on daily life, affecting social, emotional, and physical well-being. On the physical side, the chronic pain and fatigue that accompany these conditions can make everyday tasks difficult, like walking, cooking, or even getting out of bed.

This can result in a loss of independence and the need for assistance with daily activities, which can negatively impact one's sense of autonomy.

Because autoimmune diseases are unpredictable with frequent flare-ups and remissions, living with a chronic illness can be emotionally taxing and can result in feelings of frustration, anxiety, and depression. This emotional toll can exacerbate physical symptoms, creating a vicious cycle that is difficult to break without comprehensive medical and psychological support.

The social consequences of autoimmune diseases can include social distancing, diminished quality of life, and difficulty engaging in social activities, sustaining relationships, and carrying out work or family obligations due to physical and emotional constraints. These effects can be lessened with the assistance of support groups, counseling, and skillful communication with friends and family, which create a network of understanding and support for individuals coping with autoimmune conditions.

DIET IS IMPORTANT FOR MANAGING SYMPTOMS

Understanding and avoiding trigger foods is a key strategy in managing autoimmune conditions. Common triggers include gluten, dairy, and processed foods, which can increase inflammation and worsen symptoms. Diet plays a critical role in managing the symptoms of autoimmune diseases. Certain foods can trigger inflammation and exacerbate symptoms, while others can help reduce inflammation and promote overall health.

On the other hand, foods high in antioxidants, like berries and leafy greens, help reduce oxidative stress and inflammation in the body; omega-3 fatty acids, found in fish, flaxseeds, and walnuts, have been shown to have anti-inflammatory properties, making them beneficial for individuals with autoimmune diseases. Conversely, an anti-inflammatory diet rich in fruits, vegetables, lean proteins, and healthy fats can help manage autoimmune symptoms.

A balanced diet also contributes to overall health and well-being by giving the body the nutrients it needs to function at its best. This includes making sure the body gets enough vitamins and minerals, like vitamin D, which is important for immune function. Consulting a nutritionist or dietitian can help people create a customized eating plan that promotes their health and effectively manages their autoimmune symptoms.

THE AUTOIMMUNE PROTOCOL (AIP) DIET: AN OVERVIEW

An extension of the paleo diet, the Autoimmune Protocol (AIP) Diet focuses on nutrient-dense foods and eliminates potential inflammatory triggers.

The diet is divided into several phases, with the first being an elimination phase that involves removing foods known to cause inflammation, such as grains, legumes, dairy, processed foods, and certain vegetables like nightshades. The AIP Diet is a specialized diet meant to reduce inflammation, heal the gut, and manage symptoms of autoimmune diseases.

The elimination phase typically lasts a few weeks to several months, depending on individual response and symptom improvement, and emphasizes the consumption of nutrient-dense foods such as fruits, lean meats, vegetables (except nightshades), and healthy fats. Because bone broth, fermented foods, and organ meats have a high nutrient content and may support gut health, they are also encouraged.

Following the phase of elimination, foods are progressively brought back one at a time to determine which foods cause symptoms. This process is vital to determine individual food sensitivities and customize the diet to meet specific needs.

The ultimate objective of the AIP Diet is to effectively manage autoimmune symptoms, reduce inflammation, and promote healing to help people improve their quality of life and overall health.

CHAPTER TWO

THE AIP DIET'S SCIENCE BASIS

ADVANTAGES FOR ANTI-INFLAMMATORY

To help calm the body's immune response, the Autoimmune Protocol (AIP) diet eliminates foods that may cause inflammation, such as grains, legumes, dairy, and processed sugars. Instead, it emphasizes nutrient-rich, anti-inflammatory foods like fruits, vegetables, lean meats, and healthy fats.

These foods provide antioxidants and other compounds that help reduce inflammation, promote healing, and alleviate symptoms.

Anti-inflammatory foods are ones that you can include in your diet right away. Leafy greens like spinach and kale, berries like blueberries and strawberries, and fatty fish like salmon are good options because they are high in omega-3 fatty acids, vitamins, and minerals that work against inflammation at the cellular level. People who follow the AIP diet will notice a noticeable decrease in joint pain, skin flare-ups, and other inflammatory symptoms when they regularly consume these foods.

Maintaining a varied and balanced diet is key to maximizing the anti-inflammatory effects. Eating a variety of fruits, vegetables, and protein sources guarantees that you get a wide range of nutrients. Reducing inflammation over time also supports overall health and well-being. Furthermore, avoiding known inflammatory triggers like trans fats and refined sugars helps maintain the anti-inflammatory effects.

IMPROVEMENT IN GUT HEALTH

The AIP diet is a very effective way to support gut health, which is important for managing autoimmune diseases. It does this by removing foods that can harm the gut lining, like gluten, dairy, and legumes, and by emphasizing foods that support gut integrity and repair. AIP staples include fermented vegetables, bone broth, and plant foods high in fiber, which provide vital nutrients that support gut microbiome health and aid in healing.

Incorporating foods that promote the growth of beneficial bacteria is a key component of healing the gut. Probiotics found in fermented foods, such as kimchi, sauerkraut, and kombucha, balance the gut flora, while prebiotic foods, like garlic, onions, and asparagus, supply the fuel these bacteria need to grow. This symbiotic relationship between probiotics and prebiotics is essential for gut health restoration and immune system function enhancement.

In addition to the gut-friendly foods found in the AIP diet, mindful eating practices are crucial for supporting gut health. Eating mindfully means chewing food thoroughly, eating slowly, and drinking plenty of water. These small but powerful changes in digestion and nutrient absorption can have a big impact on people's digestive health and ultimately improve their overall health.

MODULATION OF THE IMMUNE SYSTEM

The main objective of the AIP diet is to balance and modulate the immune system. It does this by eliminating foods that can cause an immune response, like nightshades, grains, and legumes. This lowers the body's autoimmune activity and helps to stabilize the immune system over time by emphasizing foods that are less likely to cause an immune response.

Foods like fatty fish, avocados, and berries are packed with nutrients that support immune health, including omega-3 fatty acids, vitamins C and E, and zinc. These nutrients play a critical role in regulating immune function, reducing the severity of autoimmune responses, and promoting overall immune balance. Key foods that support immune modulation include lean proteins, healthy fats, and a variety of fruits and vegetables.

To bolster immune modulation even more, it's advantageous to incorporate immune-regulating herbs and spices (green tea, turmeric, and ginger are great options that are simple to incorporate into meals and drinks). These natural compounds have antioxidant and anti-inflammatory qualities that aid in immune modulation, offering extra support to individuals following the AIP diet.

EMPHASIS ON NUTRIENT DENSITY

Focusing on whole, unprocessed foods, the AIP diet offers a rich array of nutrients that support overall health and healing. By emphasizing nutrient density, which ensures that every bite is packed with essential vitamins, minerals, and phytonutrients, this approach helps to address potential nutrient deficiencies often seen in individuals with autoimmune diseases.

To achieve nutrient density, it is essential to include a variety of colorful vegetables, fruits, and high-quality proteins. Leafy greens, cruciferous vegetables, and vibrantly colored fruits, such as citrus and berries, are excellent sources of essential nutrients. These foods also contain high concentrations of folate, magnesium, potassium, and vitamins A, C, and K, all of which are vital for promoting health and supporting the body's healing processes.

Nutrient-dense animal products are another important way to maximize intake of nutrients. Rich in iron, B12, and A, organ meats like liver are especially beneficial. Omega-3 fatty acids and trace minerals like zinc and selenium can be found in shellfish and fatty fish.

By incorporating these nutrient-dense foods into the AIP diet, people can make sure they are getting the nutrients they need while also assisting their body's natural healing processes.

STUDIES ABOUT THE AIP DIET

An increasing amount of research is demonstrating how well the AIP diet works in treating autoimmune diseases. This includes studies that highlight the diet's capacity to lower inflammation, enhance gut health, and modulate the immune system, as well as how well it can significantly improve symptoms and quality of life for people with conditions like rheumatoid arthritis, inflammatory bowel disease, and Hashimoto's thyroiditis.

The AIP diet has been shown to reduce markers of inflammation and autoimmune activity in participants in clinical trials; for instance, a study on people with inflammatory bowel disease found that the AIP diet significantly improved clinical symptoms and quality of life; another study on patients with Hashimoto's thyroiditis reported reductions in thyroid antibodies and improvements in overall well-being.

An abundance of personal accounts, coupled with scientific research, affirm the AIP diet's potential as a potent tool for managing autoimmune diseases and enhancing general health. Numerous individuals who have followed the diet report significant improvements in their overall health, including a decrease in pain, fatigue, and other incapacitating symptoms.

CHAPTER THREE

FOODS TO ADD

Start with a variety of vegetables, such as leafy greens, cruciferous veggies like broccoli and cauliflower, and root vegetables like sweet potatoes and carrots. These provide essential vitamins, minerals, and fiber, which are crucial for gut health.

Also, include fruits like berries, apples, and bananas in moderation to benefit from their natural sweetness and antioxidants. Nutrient-dense, whole foods are the focus of the AIP diet, helping to reduce inflammation and support healing.

Another essential element of the AIP diet is protein. Choose high-quality sources like pasture-raised poultry, wild-caught fish, and grass-fed meats. Organ meats are not usually included in diets, but they are extremely nutrient-dense and can be beneficial if consumed regularly.

Bone broth is a staple of the AIP diet because of its gut-healing qualities. Try to incorporate a range of these protein sources to keep your meals interesting and nutritionally balanced.

Incorporating healthy fats into your meals will ensure you're getting enough calories and supporting your body's healing process. Avocados, coconut oil, and olive oil are great options that can help reduce inflammation and provide sustained energy. Coconut products, like coconut milk and coconut flour, are versatile and can be used in many AIP-friendly recipes.

ITEMS TO STEER CLEAR OF

Legumes, such as beans, lentils, and peanuts, should also be avoided as they contain compounds that can interfere with nutrient absorption and promote inflammation. Dairy products are excluded because they can be inflammatory for many people with autoimmune conditions. Inflammatory foods, such as wheat, rice, and oats, are prohibited on the AIP diet because they have the potential to irritate the gut lining.

AIP diet avoidance also includes avoiding nightshade vegetables (tomatoes, potatoes, eggplants, and peppers) because they contain alkaloids, which can cause inflammation in sensitive people.

Nuts and seeds are generally regarded as healthy, but they are not allowed because they can cause immune reactions and gut irritation. You should also be aware of hidden sources of these ingredients in processed foods and restaurant dishes.

The AIP diet strictly prohibits processed foods and refined sugars, which can cause blood sugar imbalances, inflammation, and nutrient deficiencies. Rather than focusing on processed foods, you should emphasize whole, unprocessed foods to support your body's healing.

By removing these inflammatory foods, you can help your immune system reset and lessen the severity of autoimmune symptoms.

TIPS FOR MEAL PLANNING

The secret to successfully implementing the AIP diet is effective meal planning. To start, make a weekly meal plan that consists of a variety of AIP-compliant foods to ensure nutritional balance. For breakfast, consider nutrient-dense smoothies with greens and fruit, or use leftover protein and vegetables from dinner. For lunch and dinner, consider simple, balanced dishes like grilled meats with roasted vegetables and a side salad. Experimenting with different colors and textures will keep your meals interesting and fulfilling.

An easy way to plan meals on the AIP diet is to batch cook. Take a few hours on the weekend to prepare a large amount of proteins, veggies, and bone broth, then store them in the refrigerator or freezer for easy access during the week. This way, you'll always have options that are AIP-friendly, which will make it easier to stick to the diet even on hectic days. To stave off hunger, you can also prepare snacks like vegetable sticks, fruit, and homemade AIP-compliant bars.

When you plan and prepare in bulk, you'll find it easier to stick to the AIP diet and enjoy a variety of delicious, healing foods. For example, roast a whole chicken and use the meat in various dishes throughout the week, such as salads, soups, and stir-fries. Keep a list of your favorite AIP recipes and rotate them to prevent meal fatigue.

Making a thorough shopping list is crucial when getting ready to start the AIP diet. Start with fresh produce, focusing on seasonal and organic products when you can. A wide range of leafy greens, cruciferous vegetables, root vegetables, and low-sugar fruits, such as berries, should be on your list because they will provide the essential vitamins and antioxidants for your meals and snacks.

Another important item on your shopping list is protein sources. Look for organ meats, wild-caught fish, pasture-raised poultry, and grass-fed beef. You should also include ingredients for bone broth, like organic vegetables and the bones of grass-fed animals. Having these proteins on hand will guarantee that you can make satiating, nutrient-rich meals. You should also stock up on canned or frozen fish, like salmon and sardines, for easy and quick options.

Stock your kitchen with healthy fats and pantry staples, such as avocados, coconut oil, olive oil, and coconut products like flour and milk; these items work well in many different recipes. For extra taste and health benefits, add fresh herbs, garlic, and ginger to your list. Having these items in your pantry will also make it easier to make AIP-compliant meals and snacks.

HOW TO GET YOUR KITCHEN READY FOR AIP

Getting your pantry and fridge clear of any non-compliant foods that could tempt you to stray from the diet is the first step in preparing your kitchen for the AIP diet. You can donate any unopened items to a local food bank or give them to friends and family. A clean, organized space will help you concentrate on your AIP journey.

A good chef's knife, cutting board, and sturdy cookware are essential for preparing AIP meals. If you're looking to cut down on cooking time and simplify the process, consider getting an Instant Pot or slow cooker; these appliances are great for making bone broth, soups, and stews. Keeping storage containers on hand will also help you keep leftovers and batch-cooked meals fresh and accessible.

Designate a space in your kitchen for meal prep and cooking. Arrange your supplies and equipment so that they are easily accessible. Stock up on a variety of herbs and spices to flavor your food. Print off AIP-friendly recipes and store them in a binder for easy access. By successfully organizing your kitchen, you'll create a setting that supports your success on the AIP diet, making it simpler to follow the plan and reap the rewards of better health.

CHAPTER FOUR

MAKING THE SWITCH TO THE AIP DIET

TRANSITIONING GRADUALLY VERSUS IMMEDIATELY

There are two ways to transition to the AIP diet: gradual or immediate. With a gradual transition, you gradually cut out non-compliant foods over a few weeks or months, giving your body time to adjust to the new eating habits. For example, you could start by cutting out dairy and grains for the first two weeks, then move on to removing legumes and nightshades in the next weeks. This is a good option for people who prefer a more manageable pace and don't find the idea of an abrupt overhaul intimidating.

An immediate transition, on the other hand, entails eliminating all non-compliant foods at once. This method can be difficult, but it can also yield quicker results. It requires careful planning, including meal planning and stockpiling AIP-compliant foods in your pantry.

Immediate transitions may work well for people who are highly motivated and prepared to dedicate themselves fully to the diet right away. It's important to mentally prepare yourself for the first few weeks of the adjustment period, which can include intense cravings and withdrawal symptoms as your body adjusts to the new eating pattern.

Both approaches require a commitment to learning new recipes, deciphering food labels, and possibly handling social situations involving food. Speaking with a healthcare provider or a nutritionist experienced in AIP can offer additional support and guidance, ensuring that the transition is seamless and catered to your particular health needs. Regardless of the approach you choose, it's important to listen to your body and be patient with yourself.

HANDLING WITHDRAWALS AND CRAVINGS

A key component of making the switch to the AIP diet is learning how to deal with cravings and withdrawals.

When your body cleanses from sugar, caffeine, and processed foods, you may have strong cravings as well as withdrawal symptoms like headaches, fatigue, and irritability. To help you deal with these symptoms, concentrate on eating foods high in nutrients that will satisfy your hunger and reduce cravings. You should also include plenty of protein, healthy fats, and vegetables high in fiber to keep your blood sugar stable and prevent hunger pangs.

Another important tactic for controlling cravings is to stay hydrated. Often, what we think of as hunger or cravings is dehydration, so drinking lots of water throughout the day can help alleviate these sensations. Herbal teas and bone broths can also be calming and provide essential nutrients. You can also distract yourself from cravings by walking, reading, or doing something fun.

Maintaining a food journal to document your triggers and responses can also offer insightful information and help you stay on track. Supportive practices like mindful eating and stress-reduction methods like yoga or meditation can further assist in managing cravings and withdrawals. These practices can improve your relationship with food and enhance your overall well-being.

LOCATING RESOURCES AND ASSISTANCE

A successful transition to the AIP diet requires finding resources and support. Local support groups or workshops can also offer a sense of community and face-to-face interaction. Reaching out to others who are following the AIP diet can provide motivation, encouragement, and useful advice. Online communities, such as forums and social media groups, can be invaluable for sharing experiences, recipes, and tips.

Several authors and bloggers specialize in the AIP diet and offer free guides, cookbooks, and shopping lists. These resources can make meal planning easier and guarantee you have a variety of tasty and compliant options to choose from.

Other crucial steps in staying on track include keeping a well-stocked pantry with AIP staples and learning how to read food labels. Books, blogs, and websites dedicated to the AIP diet can be excellent resources for recipes, meal plans, and scientific information.

To meet your nutritional needs while managing your autoimmune condition, it can be helpful to have professional support from a healthcare provider, such as a nutritionist or dietitian experienced in AIP. They can offer personalized guidance and address any specific health concerns, as well as help you create a balanced meal plan, monitor your progress, and make necessary dietary adjustments.

MONITORING YOUR DEVELOPMENT

Monitoring your progress on the AIP diet is critical to comprehending the impact of the dietary modifications on your health. Maintaining a thorough food journal can assist you in recognizing trends and connections between your eating habits and your emotional state.

Record the foods you eat, any symptoms you encounter, and other pertinent variables such as stress levels and sleep patterns. This data can be extremely helpful in identifying food triggers and assisting you in modifying your diet.

Monitoring objective health markers (weight, blood pressure, lab results) regularly can help you see improvements in your health that may not be immediately apparent. Tracking subjective health markers (pain relief, increased energy, improved mood) can also help you stay motivated and committed to the diet by helping you think back on these positive changes and reinforce the benefits of following the AIP protocol.

Tracking your progress not only helps you fine-tune your diet but also serves as a powerful reminder of how far you've come on your health journey. Using apps or digital tools designed for diet tracking can make this process easier and more efficient. Many apps offer features specifically for people with dietary restrictions, allowing you to log your meals and symptoms conveniently. Sharing your progress with a healthcare provider or support group can provide additional accountability and encouragement.

HAVING REASONABLE OBJECTIVES

A key to successfully implementing the AIP diet is setting realistic goals. Begin by identifying your overall goals, such as managing an autoimmune condition, reducing specific symptoms, or improving general health. Then, break these big goals down into smaller, more doable tasks. For example, if your goal is to reduce joint pain, a smaller goal might be to regularly eat anti-inflammatory foods and stay away from known triggers for a month.

To help you stay focused and track your progress more effectively, make sure your goals are specific, measurable, attainable, relevant, and time-bound (SMART). You should also be flexible and adjust your goals as needed based on your body's responses and any new insights you gain along the way. Instead of setting a vague goal like "feel better," aim for something more concrete, like "reduce joint pain by 50% in three months."

Remember, transitioning to the AIP diet is a journey that requires patience and persistence. By setting realistic goals and steadily working towards them, you can achieve long-lasting improvements in your health and well-being. Honor your efforts and the progress you've made, no matter how minor it may seem. This positive reinforcement can boost your morale and encourage you to continue adhering to the diet.

CHAPTER FIVE

PLANNING AND PREPARING MEALS

WEEKLY GUIDE TO MEAL PLANNING

Weekly meal planning is a key component of the Autoimmune Protocol (AIP) diet. To begin, set aside some time on the weekends to plan your meals for the coming week. This involves choosing recipes that are compliant with the AIP and making sure they don't contain any inflammatory ingredients, such as grains, dairy, legumes, or nightshades. You can use an app or calendar to schedule your meals, and make sure your breakfast, lunch, and dinner include a variety of proteins, vegetables, and healthy fats. By organizing your meals ahead of time, you can minimize last-minute stress and stay on track with your dietary objectives.

Next, make a thorough shopping list based on your meal plan. Having a thorough list will make grocery shopping easier and prevent you from making unwarranted purchases. Local farmers' markets offer fresh, organic produce and meats that are perfect for the AIP diet. You can also stock up on pantry staples like bone broth, coconut oil, and AIP-compliant seasonings to add flavor and nutrition to your meals.

To ensure that cooking during the week is quick and easy, reduce the temptation to stray from your diet due to time constraints or lack of ingredients. Lastly, prep as much as you can ahead of time. Wash, chop, and store vegetables in airtight containers. Marinate proteins to enhance their flavor. Pre-portion snacks like carrot sticks or apple slices to grab on the go.

BATCH COOKING AND PREPARING MEALS

Batch cooking is a great way to stick to an AIP diet with little daily work. To start, choose a day of the week, usually Sunday, and spend a lot of time making large amounts of AIP-compliant meals that can be frozen and eaten throughout the week. You should concentrate on making recipes that are easy to reheat and eat again, like soups, stews, and casseroles.

You should also buy good storage containers to keep your meals organized and fresh.

Cook proteins in bulk during your batch cooking session: roast a few chicken breasts, bake a big piece of fish, or make a big batch of ground turkey or beef. Cook a variety of vegetables at the same time: roast sweet potatoes, steam broccoli, and sauté leafy greens. Portion these foods into containers and mix and match the proteins and vegetables to make balanced meals that you can quickly prepare by just grabbing a container.

To make life even easier, think about preparing breakfast and snacks in advance. Bake some AIP muffins or make a big pot of AIP-friendly porridge. Make smoothie packs by slicing fruits and veggies into freezer bags so you can whip up a healthy breakfast in the morning. Having snacks on hand, such as jerky, boiled eggs, or AIP energy bites, will help you stay full and on track with your diet all day.

With a little imagination, breakfast on the AIP diet can be tasty and nourishing. To start your day off right, make a filling AIP smoothie by blending coconut milk, a few berries, a scoop of collagen protein, and some greens, such as spinach or kale.

This smoothie is full of nutrients and makes a convenient, quick, and portable breakfast option. To add some variation to your morning smoothies, try combining different fruits and vegetables.

A sweet potato hash is another great AIP breakfast option. Dice the sweet potatoes and sauté them with onions, garlic, and your preferred AIP-compliant herbs and spices.

For protein, add some ground turkey or leftover roast chicken, and top with a big handful of fresh greens, like spinach or kale. This hash is flavorful, filling, and easy to prepare ahead of time for hectic mornings.

AIP-compliant muffins can be a satisfying replacement for traditional baked goods. The base of these muffins is made of coconut flour, ripe bananas, and unsweetened applesauce. For flavor and texture, you can add in blueberries or grated zucchini. Bake a batch on the weekend and have these muffins for breakfast or as a quick snack throughout the week. This way, you'll always have a satisfying and compliant option on hand when hunger strikes.

EASY AIP LUNCH RECIPES

The key to making easy and fulfilling AIP lunches is to combine fresh ingredients with minimal preparation. A light and nutrient-dense salad is a great starting point; start with a bed of mixed greens and top with vibrant veggies like sliced cucumbers, grilled chicken, or salmon. Drizzle with an easy AIP-friendly dressing made of olive oil, lemon juice, and herbs.

Salad wraps are another simple and quick lunch option. Take large, sturdy lettuce leaves, such as butter or romaine, and roll them out.

Stuff them with cooked ground meat, diced avocado, and shredded vegetables; top with fresh cilantro and a squeeze of lime for extra flavor. These wraps are adaptable, so you can switch up the fillings to keep things interesting while following the AIP guidelines.

Try this easy bone broth soup for a hearty and satisfying midday meal. Start with a base of homemade or store-bought AIP-compliant bone broth, then add cooked vegetables like carrots, celery, and zucchini. Add shredded chicken or beef for protein, and season with garlic, ginger, and fresh herbs. This soup can be made in big batches and then reheated for a healthy and easy weekday meal.

SCRUMPTIOUS AIP DINNER IDEAS

With the right recipes, AIP dinners can be flavorful and satisfying. One such recipe is a classic roasted chicken and vegetable medley. To make this dish, season a whole chicken with herbs and spices that are friendly to the AIP and roast it alongside a mixture of root vegetables, such as carrots, parsnips, and sweet potatoes. The chicken will stay juicy and flavorful while the vegetables will get tender and caramelized, creating a satisfying and well-balanced supper.

Another delicious AIP dinner option is a flavorful stir-fry. To make it AIP-compliant and add some nice texture, use coconut oil to sauté thinly sliced beef or chicken with a variety of vegetables, such as bell peppers, broccoli, and snap peas. Season with ginger, garlic, and a dash of coconut aminos for a savory and satisfying dish. Serve over cauliflower rice.

Shepherd's pie is a delicious and AIP-compliant dinner that can be made ahead of time and reheated to ensure you have a wholesome, comforting meal ready when you need it. Start by using ground lamb or beef for the base, cooking it with onions, carrots, and celery until it becomes tender. Top with a creamy mash made from steamed and blended cauliflower or sweet potatoes. Bake until golden and bubbly.

RECIPES THAT FOLLOW THE AIP DIET

BREAKFAST RECIPES

Begin your day with filling and delectable options that follow the Autoimmune Protocol (AIP) diet. An AIP breakfast typically consists of nutrient-dense ingredients like sweet potatoes, greens, and mildly digestible protein sources. Take into account recipes like AIP-friendly smoothie bowls that combine coconut milk, berries, and collagen protein for long-lasting energy. Alternatively, bake sweet potato hash browns with avocado slices and a side of nitrate-free bacon for a substantial morning meal. These recipes not only accommodate your dietary restrictions but also guarantee that you start your day with a balanced diet that helps manage your autoimmune symptoms.

LUNCH AND DINNER RECIPES

An AIP diet that emphasizes lean proteins, healthy fats, and a variety of vegetables will provide you with satisfying lunch and dinner options.

For example, a flavorful and filling main course could be grilled lemon herb chicken served alongside roasted root vegetables, like carrots and parsnips. Alternatively, you could try a nourishing AIP-friendly soup, like butternut squash soup seasoned with turmeric and ginger, served alongside a mixed green salad dressed in avocado and olive oil dressing.

These recipes emphasize whole foods and steer clear of common inflammatory triggers, which makes them ideal for supporting autoimmune health while enjoying satisfying meals throughout the day.

SNACKS AND DESSERT RECIPES

Nourish your hunger in between meals with wholesome AIP-approved snacks and indulge in guilt-free desserts. Try kale chips seasoned with sea salt and nutritional yeast as a snack, or make your trail mix with dried fruits and coconut flakes. For dessert, try coconut milk-based berry sorbet or baked cinnamon apples drenched in coconut butter.

These snack and dessert ideas are not only AIP compliant but also offer delicious substitutes for traditional snacks and sweets.

Refresh yourself and your body with nutrient-dense, AIP-compliant smoothies and drinks. For example, whip up a tropical green smoothie with coconut water, spinach, pineapple, and cucumber for a hydrating, nutrient-dense drink. Or, savor a creamy avocado and banana smoothie made with coconut milk and a dash of vanilla extract for a delightful treat.

For warm beverages, think about herbal teas like ginger turmeric tea or a calming bone broth infused with herbs and vegetables. These smoothies and drinks not only improve your hydration but also supply vital vitamins and minerals that boost your immune system and general health.

To maintain dietary restrictions while still enjoying rich flavors, consider cooking a slow-cooked beef stew with root vegetables and fresh herbs for a cozy family gathering. These tasty and festive meal ideas highlight the versatility of the AIP diet, providing comforting and satisfying dishes that everyone can enjoy together while supporting optimal health and well-being. For example, prepare a herb-crusted roast turkey served with cauliflower mash and roasted Brussels sprouts for a delicious holiday feast.

Whether you're starting your day with a nutrient-packed breakfast, enjoying satisfying lunches and dinners, indulging in snacks and desserts, staying hydrated with smoothies and drinks, or celebrating special occasions, these recipes and meal ideas show how the Autoimmune Protocol can be used in real life to make sure that every meal is not only nutritious but also delicious and simple to prepare.

SIMPLE AND QUICK SNACK IDEAS

Snacking on the AIP diet can be tasty and fulfilling. One of the easiest snacks to make is sliced apples with a homemade coconut butter drizzle, which is made simply by blending unsweetened shredded coconut until it becomes creamy. This combination provides both a sweet treat and healthy fats and fiber.

Another simple snack is a handful of mixed berries sprinkled with shredded coconut, which is refreshing and full of antioxidants, making it ideal for a quick energy boost.

Another healthy snack that's easy to prep ahead of time is a container of chopped carrots, celery, cucumbers, and bell peppers. These crunchy veggies go well with homemade guacamole or a wholesome avocado, lime juice, and sea salt dip. Both of these dips are nutrient-dense, so they'll keep you full and nourished in between meals.

Plantain chips can also be a great substitute for regular potato chips. Just thinly slice the plantains, toss them in olive oil, and bake until crispy for a salty, crunchy snack.

If you're in the mood for something a little bit more protein-heavy, try these portable snacks: AIP-compliant beef jerky or turkey rolls, which are made by seasoning thinly sliced meat with herbs and baking on low heat until dry. These are great for busy days and offer a good source of protein to keep you energized. To make the rolls, simply wrap slices of turkey around cucumber sticks or avocado slices.

NUTRITIOUS AIP DESSERTS

With a little imagination, it's possible to enjoy desserts while following the AIP diet. One easy and delightful recipe is coconut milk chia pudding, which is made by combining chia seeds with coconut milk and refrigerating it overnight. The next morning, you'll have a creamy pudding that tastes great and is high in fiber and omega-3 fatty acids. You can even top it with fresh berries or a sprinkle of cinnamon.

Another simple and healthful AIP dessert is banana ice cream, which is made by freezing ripe bananas and then blending them until they are smooth and creamy. You can add chocolate flavoring by adding carob powder, or you can add sweetness by mixing in some fresh berries. This dessert is great for satisfying your sweet tooth without going overboard with AIP guidelines. You can also make baked apple slices by slicing apples, dusting them with cinnamon, and baking them until they are soft. You can serve these with a dollop of coconut cream for a warm and comforting dessert.

Baking enthusiasts can make AIP-compliant cookies with coconut flour, coconut oil, and a natural sweetener such as honey or maple syrup. Toss in some dried fruit or carob chips for flavor and bake until golden brown. These cookies are a great way to enjoy a sweet treat without having to use any of the inflammatory ingredients that are present in traditional desserts.

They're also a healthier option that fits well with the AIP diet.

OPTIONS FOR PORTABLE SNACKS

Making your trail mix is a great way to keep your diet on track when you're on the go. Dried fruit, such as figs or apricots, can be combined with tiger nuts and coconut flakes to create a crunchy, sweet snack that's easy to pack and delivers a good balance of natural sugars, fats, and fiber to keep you full throughout the day.

AIP-compliant energy balls are yet another delicious and portable snack. Simply blend dates, shredded coconut, and a small amount of coconut oil; roll into bite-sized balls and refrigerate.

Energy balls are a great way to fuel up quickly and are high in nutrients and healthy fats. You can even add different flavorings, like vanilla extract or carob powder, to keep them interesting.

Meat sticks and jerky are also great on-the-go snacks. You can make your own by marinating strips of beef or turkey in a mixture of coconut aminos, garlic, and herbs, and then drying them. These high-protein snacks are easy to carry, so they're great for long days or trips. Pair them with some fresh fruit or veggie sticks for a satisfying and well-balanced snack that you can eat anywhere.

HOW TO MAKE YOUR AIP SWEETS

Making your own AIP treats gives you total control over the flavors and ingredients, so you can indulge your cravings while adhering to the diet. Start with easy recipes like homemade fruit leather, which is a lot of fun to make and is great for both kids and adults. Simply puree your favorite fruits, spread the mixture thinly on a baking sheet, and dehydrate it in the oven. Once dried, cut the mixture into strips for a naturally sweet and chewy snack.

AIP granola is another delicious homemade treat. Combine shredded coconut, chopped dried fruit, and tiger nuts with a small amount of coconut oil and honey. Bake until golden brown and crunchy. This granola is delicious on its own, with coconut yogurt, or as a fruit topping. It has a satisfying crunch and a flavorful burst, making it a versatile snack option. AIP muffins made with coconut flour, ripe bananas, and applesauce can also be moist and delicious. For added flavor, add blueberries or carob chips.

A savory alternative would be to make AIP-compliant crackers: just mix cassava flour, olive oil, and herbs; roll out the dough and bake until crisp; these crackers have a nice crunch and go well with guacamole or other compliant dips. You can customize the flavors and ingredients to your taste preferences when you make your treats.

MAINTAINING CONTENTMENT BETWEEN MEALS

The AIP diet allows you to maintain your energy and nutrient levels between meals, so you can stay fuller between meals. You can prevent hunger pangs by including protein-dense snacks like turkey slices or boiled eggs, which are simple to prepare ahead of time and can be refrigerated for easy access. You can also serve boiled eggs with some fresh vegetables or fruit for a well-balanced mini-meal.

The healthy fats in avocados help maintain satiety and provide essential nutrients; similarly, a handful of olives or a small serving of coconut yogurt with a drizzle of honey can offer a satisfying combination of fats and natural sugars, helping to stabilize blood sugar levels and prevent energy dips. Additionally, avocado slices sprinkled with sea salt and a dash of lime juice make a delicious and filling snack.

High-fiber snacks like fresh fruits and vegetables can help you feel fuller for longer. Apple slices, carrot sticks, or a small salad with mixed greens and a light olive oil dressing can be nourishing and filling. Fiber slows down digestion and keeps your energy level constant, so it's a must for between-meal snacks.

CHAPTER SIX

IDENTIFYING RESTAURANTS THAT ACCEPT AIP

Finding restaurants that can meet your dietary requirements when dining out on the AIP diet can be difficult, but it is doable with some planning and research. Look for restaurants that offer farm-to-table, paleo, or gluten-free options; these establishments are more likely to be aware of and accommodating of AIP restrictions.

Use apps and online resources devoted to special diets to find reviews and recommendations for AIP-friendly restaurants in your area. If in doubt, give the restaurant a call in advance to ask if they can alter their menu items to meet your dietary requirements.

Once you are at the restaurant, carefully go through the menu and look for simple, whole-food-based dishes like grilled meats, fish, and vegetable sides. Avoid anything that contains grains, dairy, legumes, or nightshades.

Salads are a great option a lot of the time, but make sure the dressings and toppings are compliant by asking about the ingredients or asking for oil and vinegar on the side. Don't be afraid to ask the waiter detailed questions about how the dishes are prepared and if any modifications can be made to meet your needs.

Furthermore, be ready to substitute ingredients or make other AIP-friendly dish modifications. For instance, ask to have your protein grilled without seasonings or marinades, or request steamed veggies rather than fried or sautéed ones. A lot of restaurants are accommodating to dietary needs as long as you are upfront and courteous about your needs. Being proactive and prepared will allow you to enjoy dining out without sacrificing your AIP diet.

SHARING YOUR NUTRITIONAL REQUIREMENTS

When dining out on the AIP diet, it is important to communicate your dietary needs clearly and concisely. Begin by outlining exactly what you can and cannot eat, along with a brief description of the foods you must avoid, including grains, dairy, legumes, nuts, seeds, nightshades, and processed foods. This will help the restaurant staff understand how important your dietary needs are.

A polite request to learn more about the preparation of the dishes and suggestions for menu items that can be changed to suit your diet should be made when discussing your dietary requirements with the waiter or chef.

Be specific about substitutions, like asking for steamed vegetables instead of rice or olive oil in place of butter, and the kitchen staff will be able to better accommodate your needs if you provide them with clear instructions.

Clear communication is key to having a pleasant dining experience while adhering to the AIP diet. You can also carry a dining card that outlines your dietary restrictions. This card can be given to the waiter to relay to the chef, preventing any misunderstanding about your needs.

You can also prepare a brief explanation of your diet to avoid long discussions at the table, keeping the dining experience enjoyable for everyone involved.

HOW TO TRAVEL WITH AIP MEALS AND SNACKS

The secret to traveling on the AIP diet and having access to compliant meals and snacks is to prepare ahead of time. Start by packing a variety of AIP-friendly snacks, like dehydrated fruits, nuts, and homemade jerky; these are easy to carry and can provide you with a quick source of nutrition when you're on the go. You should also think about packing and preparing meals that travel well, like roasted vegetables, grilled chicken, and simple salads; use insulated containers to keep these meals fresh and ready to eat.

Make a list of the things you'll need, like fresh produce, organic meats, and compliant condiments, and before you leave, research your destination to find markets and grocery stores that sell AIP-friendly foods. Many health food stores and larger supermarkets carry a variety of organic and natural products that fit within the AIP guidelines. If you have access to a kitchen while traveling, make plans to cook some of your meals to make sure they meet your dietary needs.

Having a plan in place for both dining out and cooking for yourself will help you stick to the AIP diet while traveling. In addition to packing your food, be ready for situations where you might need to eat out. Research nearby restaurants that offer AIP-friendly options or are willing to accommodate dietary restrictions. Call ahead to inquire about their menu and any possible modifications.

SOME ADVICE FOR MAINTAINING FOCUS WHILE TRAVELING

Making a list of AIP-friendly foods and snacks to pack in advance will help you prioritize your health and stay on track with your diet while on vacation. Make sure your list includes a variety of portable options, such as fresh fruits, vegetables, and pre-cooked proteins, to keep you satisfied and energized throughout your trip. First, set realistic goals for your trip, acknowledging that some flexibility may be necessary.

Look for simple dishes with whole food ingredients and steer clear of processed or fried foods. When dining out, do your homework in advance and find restaurants that are willing to accommodate your dietary needs or offer AIP-friendly options. Don't be afraid to ask questions about menu items and request modifications to ensure your meals are compliant. Remember that many restaurants are willing to make adjustments if you communicate your needs clearly and politely.

Consistency and mindfulness will help you enjoy your vacation while staying true to your dietary goals. Managing temptations and remaining mindful of your choices will help you stick to your AIP diet while on vacation. Focus on the delicious, compliant foods you can enjoy to avoid feeling deprived. If you find yourself in a situation where compliant options are limited, try your best to make the healthiest choice available and get back on track with your next meal.

It can be difficult to navigate food-related social events when following the AIP diet, but it is doable with some preparation and communication. First, let the host know that you have dietary restrictions; be clear about what you need and offer to bring a dish to share that complies with the AIP diet. This will not only guarantee that you have something to eat, but it will also introduce others to AIP-friendly foods. A delicious and simple salad with a compliant dressing or roasted vegetable platter is good option.

Eat whole, unprocessed foods and steer clear of dishes that contain grains, dairy, legumes, or nightshades. Instead, opt for simple options like grilled meats, fresh vegetables, and fruits. If you're unsure about the ingredients in a particular dish, it's best to ask the host or politely decline. At the event, concentrate more on the social aspects than the food. Participate in activities, have conversations, and enjoy the company of friends and family.

Taking care of social events also means being ready for circumstances in which there may not be many compliant options. Bring some AIP-friendly snacks, like fruit or homemade jerky, so you'll always have something to eat. Remain upbeat and adaptable, concentrating on the social experience rather than the restrictions of your diet. By being prepared and clear about your needs, you can enjoy social gatherings without sacrificing your AIP diet.

CHAPTER SEVEN

HANDLING EMOTIONAL EATING AND CRAVINGS

RECOGNIZING CRAVINGS AND WHAT CAUSES THEM

An intricate web of emotional, psychological, and physiological variables frequently leads to cravings; identifying these triggers is the first step toward effectively managing them. Common triggers include boredom, stress, and particular environments, like being in a kitchen or walking by a bakery. Certain foods can also set off cravings because their high sugar or fat content activates brain reward centers, making them difficult to resist. By identifying their triggers, people can begin to develop strategies to manage and mitigate cravings.

By tracking eating patterns and identifying emotional triggers, people can become more aware of their eating habits and the emotional states that precede cravings. By doing this, they can address the underlying issues rather than just treating the symptoms of the craving.

Once triggers have been identified, it is important to understand the body's signals and distinguish between true hunger and emotional cravings. True hunger is gradual and can be satisfied with various foods, while cravings are usually sudden and specific.

To effectively manage cravings, it is important to address any underlying nutritional deficiencies. For example, a chocolate craving could be a symptom of a magnesium deficiency, whereas a desire for salty snacks could be an indication of a need for more sodium or other minerals.

A balanced diet high in essential nutrients can help lower the frequency and intensity of cravings. Speaking with a healthcare provider can offer tailored insights into nutritional needs and assist in creating a diet plan that promotes overall well-being and lowers cravings.

HEALTHY SUBSTITUTES FOR OFTEN-CRAVING FOODS

A practical way to satisfy cravings without going off course with diet plans is to find healthy substitutes for common ones. For example, fresh fruit or a small piece of dark chocolate can satisfy a sweet tooth without resorting to candy or pastries; naturally sweet foods like berries or apples can be incorporated into meals and snacks to help reduce sugar cravings; and for those who prefer creamy textures, Greek yogurt with a drizzle of honey or blended frozen bananas can mimic the mouthfeel of ice cream or pudding.

Cravings for salty snacks can be controlled by choosing healthier options such as air-popped popcorn, roasted nuts, or seeds. These have the same crunch and saltiness as processed snacks and chips, but they don't have as many calories or bad fats. Adding herbs and spices to meals also improves flavor and lessens the need for extra salt. Garlic, paprika, and cumin, for example, add flavor and satisfaction to food, reducing the need for salty snacks.

If you have cravings for fried or fatty foods, try baking, grilling, or air-frying to achieve a similar texture and flavor without the added fat.

For example, air-fried chicken or baked sweet potato fries have all the flavor and crunch of traditional fried foods but are lower in calories and unhealthy fats. You can also try different cooking methods and recipes to find satisfying substitutes that fit into a healthy diet.

TECHNIQUES FOR EMOTIONAL CONSUMPTION

Developing healthy coping mechanisms, like playing sports, learning relaxation techniques, or taking up hobbies, can provide alternative outlets for stress and emotions. Exercise, in particular, has been shown to reduce stress and improve mood, making it a beneficial strategy for those prone to emotional eating. Emotional eating is frequently a response to stress, anxiety, or other negative emotions, and addressing these underlying issues is key to managing it.

Establishing regular eating patterns and mindful eating practices is another useful tactic. Mindful eating entails scheduling regular meal times, concentrating on the eating experience, appreciating each bite, and monitoring signals of hunger and fullness.

By practicing mindfulness, people can lessen the possibility that they will eat out of emotional need rather than genuine hunger. It also fosters a positive relationship between the eater and food, viewing it as nourishment rather than a coping mechanism.

Talking to someone about emotional struggles can relieve stress and lessen the need to turn to food for comfort. Support groups and therapy can provide additional tools and strategies for managing emotional eating. Professional guidance from a nutritionist or therapist can offer personalized advice and support, helping people develop a sustainable approach to managing emotional eating and improving overall well-being. Seeking support from friends, family, or professionals can also be beneficial.

STRESS REDUCTION WITH MINDFULNESS

Techniques like progressive muscle relaxation, deep breathing, and meditation can help people stay present and calm, which reduces the impulse to eat in response to stress.

Regular mindfulness practice can increase resilience to stress and improve emotional regulation, making it easier to manage cravings and emotional eating triggers. Mindfulness practices can play a significant role in managing cravings and emotional eating by promoting awareness and reducing stress.

Incorporating mindfulness practices into daily routines can also improve the eating experience and cultivate a positive relationship with food. Mindful eating entails savoring food by paying attention to its flavor, texture, and aroma; eating slowly; and identifying cues from hunger and fullness.

Over time, mindful eating can lessen the propensity to overeat and increase awareness of the emotional and physical aspects of eating.

An individual's reliance on food as a coping mechanism can be decreased by identifying sources of stress and creating a plan to manage them. This plan may include time management techniques, realistic goal-setting and incorporating relaxation activities into daily routines.

By proactively managing stress, individuals can create a more balanced and healthy lifestyle that supports better eating habits and lowers the likelihood of emotional eating. Stress management is important for overall health and can have a significant impact on eating behaviors.

CREATING A HELPFUL ENVIRONMENT

Managing cravings and emotional eating requires a supportive environment, which begins at home with organizing the kitchen and pantry to prioritize healthy foods, stocking healthy foods and removing temptations to help you make better choices, and keeping wholesome snacks like fruits, vegetables, nuts, and whole grains handy to help you satisfy your hunger and cravings without turning to unhealthy options.

To effectively manage cravings and emotional eating, social support is essential. Connecting with friends, family, or support groups that share and comprehend dietary goals can be a source of inspiration and encouragement.

Sharing successes and setbacks with others can establish a sense of accountability and lessen feelings of loneliness. Taking part in group activities, like exercise or cooking classes, can also help to build a sense of community and offer extra support for sticking to healthy habits.

A supportive environment in all facets of life can help individuals create a framework that supports their dietary goals and makes it easier to manage cravings and emotional eating. Work and social environments can also be modified to support healthy eating. Examples of this include packing a healthy lunch for work, avoiding vending machines, and choosing restaurants with healthy options when dining out. Communicating dietary goals with colleagues and friends can help ensure that social events and gatherings offer suitable food choices.

CHAPTER EIGHT

KEEPING AN EYE ON YOUR PROGRESS AND MODIFYING YOUR DIET

MAINTAINING A FOOD AND SYMPTOM RECORD

When following an Autoimmune Protocol (AIP) diet, keeping a food and symptom journal is essential. It helps you keep track of everything you eat and any symptoms you encounter, giving you important insights into how different foods affect your body. To begin, list everything you eat throughout the day, including ingredients and portion sizes. Record the time of each meal or snack, as well as any after-effects you notice, such as bloating, fatigue, or changes in digestion. This thorough tracking allows you to identify patterns and potential triggers that could aggravate autoimmune symptoms.

To maintain an effective food and symptom journal, you should use a notebook or a specialized app that allows you to quickly enter and review your entries.

Be sure to record everything consistently and completely, as even minor details can reveal important information about how your body responds to particular foods. Review your journal entries regularly to identify patterns or connections between specific foods and symptoms.

RECOGNIZING AND BRINGING BACK FOODS

The AIP diet involves a methodical process of identifying and reintroducing foods to determine which foods might cause autoimmune responses. To start, eliminate all foods that may cause inflammation, such as grains, dairy, legumes, and vegetables from the nightshade family, for some time. Following this elimination phase, gradually reintroduce one food group at a time, beginning with the least allergenic options, like egg yolks or certain spices. During this phase, keep a close eye on your body's reactions and record any changes in symptoms or energy levels.

This systematic reintroduction process helps you better tailor your diet to your body's needs so you can enjoy a wider variety of foods while managing your autoimmune symptoms. When reintroducing foods, use an organized method to accurately identify triggers. Introduce a small portion of the food and wait for at least three days before reintroducing another type. Track your reactions in your food and symptom journal to differentiate between a normal reaction and a potential intolerance or allergy.

CHANGING THE DIET IN RESPONSE TO SYMPTOMS

A key component of managing autoimmune conditions with the AIP protocol is modifying the diet in response to symptoms. As you keep a food and symptom journal and reintroduce foods, you may notice that some foods cause persistent adverse reactions. To address this, modify your diet by eliminating or limiting these foods and placing an emphasis on nutrient-dense foods that promote healing and lower inflammation. You should also concentrate on eating a variety of fresh vegetables, high-quality proteins, and healthy fats to provide necessary nutrients without exacerbating symptoms.

Personalized advice on diet adjustments can be obtained by speaking with a healthcare professional specializing in autoimmune diseases. They can also assist in interpreting your journal entries and suggest specific dietary adjustments based on your health requirements. Dietary adjustments could involve increasing your intake of anti-inflammatory foods such as fatty fish, leafy greens, and berries, or experimenting with different cooking techniques to improve food tolerability. By making proactive dietary adjustments based on symptoms and expert advice, you can improve your health outcomes and better manage your autoimmune symptoms.

COLLABORATING WITH MEDICAL PROFESSIONALS

To effectively navigate the complexities of the AIP diet and manage autoimmune conditions, you must collaborate with a team of doctors, dietitians, and functional medicine practitioners who specialize in autoimmune diseases. This team can offer expert guidance on how to implement the AIP protocol, interpret lab results, and track your health over time. You can discuss any issues you may be having, get personalized recommendations, and modify your treatment plan at regular consultations.

Building a strong partnership with healthcare professionals ensures you receive comprehensive care, empowering you to make informed decisions and achieve sustainable improvements in your autoimmune health. They can also suggest additional therapies, such as stress management techniques, supplements, or medications, to complement your dietary efforts and optimize overall wellness. Last but not least, they can offer emotional and practical support and encouragement throughout your journey through diet changes.

HONORING ACHIEVEMENTS AND ADVANCEMENT

Maintaining motivation and sticking to the AIP diet requires celebrating progress and milestones. Set attainable goals like lowering inflammation markers, boosting energy, or improving quality of life.

Track your progress regularly using objective metrics like lab tests or subjective evaluations of the severity of your symptoms. Acknowledge and celebrate each accomplishment, no matter how big or small, like finishing a successful reintroduction phase or sticking to your diet plan in the face of difficulties.

Celebrating milestones reinforces your commitment to long-term health goals and boosts your morale, making it easier to stay motivated and resilient on your AIP journey. Share your accomplishments with supportive friends, family members, or online communities to build a positive support network. Think back on how far you've come and acknowledge the effort and dedication you've invested in improving your health. Consider rewarding yourself with non-food treats like a relaxing spa day, a new book, or an enjoyable hobby.

These synopses seek to offer concise, useful advice on all matters about tracking development and making dietary modifications in the framework of an Autoimmune Protocol Disease Cookbook.

CHAPTER NINE

ADVANCED TECHNIQUES FOR THE AIP DIET

THE USE OF FUNCTIONAL FOODS

Functional foods are high in antioxidants, anti-inflammatory compounds, and essential nutrients that support immune function and overall health. Examples of functional foods include turmeric, ginger, leafy greens, berries, and fatty fish like salmon, which are known for their omega-3 fatty acids. Functional foods also help to reduce inflammation, support gut health, and provide essential nutrients that aid in healing and managing autoimmune conditions. Including functional foods into an advanced AIP (Autoimmune Protocol) diet involves carefully choosing foods that offer therapeutic benefits beyond basic nutrition.

Aim for a rainbow of colorful fruits and vegetables to optimize nutrient intake and antioxidant benefits. Experiment with different herbs and spices known for their medicinal properties, like garlic for immune-boosting effects or cilantro for detoxification support. Source organic and local produce whenever possible to minimize pesticide exposure and maximize nutrient density. These are just a few tips for successfully incorporating functional foods into your AIP diet.

Practically speaking, begin by organizing meals that include a balance of these functional foods. For instance, prepare a nutrient-dense salad with mixed greens, colorful bell peppers, avocado, and a dressing of olive oil and lemon juice. Use protein sources such as wild-caught fish or grass-fed meats. Liberally add herbs like basil and oregano for flavor and extra health benefits. By concentrating on whole, nutrient-dense foods and creatively incorporating them into your daily meals, you can effectively harness the power of functional foods to support your autoimmune health.

TAILORED ADD-ONS

Within the framework of an advanced allergy-inflammatory protocol (AIP) diet, personalized supplementation involves adjusting dietary intake to address individual deficiencies and support optimal health outcomes. Many common allergens and irritants are restricted in the AIP diet, which can occasionally result in nutrient gaps that are filled with targeted nutrients that support immune function, gut healing, and overall well-being. Key supplements frequently include vitamin D, omega-3 fatty acids, probiotics, and specific vitamins and minerals based on individual lab tests and health assessments.

Working with a healthcare professional who is familiar with the AIP diet and autoimmune conditions is essential to successfully implementing personalized supplementation. This person can interpret lab results and suggest supplements based on your unique needs. For example, if you have low vitamin D levels, your provider may recommend a higher dose of vitamin D3 to support immune regulation and bone health. Probiotics can aid in the restoration of gut flora balance, which is critical for reducing inflammation and improving digestion—common problems in autoimmune disorders.

Personalized supplementation is a methodical approach to incorporating supplements into your daily routine. Some examples of this include creating a pill organizer, tracking any improvements in your health or changes in your symptoms, and monitoring your body's response to supplementation, making necessary adjustments under your doctor's guidance.

By tailoring your supplement regimen to your unique health needs and goals, you can improve long-term health outcomes and maximize the effectiveness of your AIP diet.

ADVANCED PROTOCOLS FOR GUT HEALING

The gut plays a major role in immune function and inflammation regulation, making it a primary area of focus in the AIP protocol. Advanced protocols often include strategies like bone broth consumption, which provides healing nutrients like collagen and amino acids that support gut lining integrity and reduce inflammation. Advanced gut healing protocols within the AIP framework focus on restoring and maintaining optimal gut health, which is crucial for managing autoimmune conditions.

Incorporating lifestyle factors like stress management techniques and adequate sleep can further support gut healing and overall immune function. Using advanced gut healing protocols also entails identifying and eliminating potential triggers that may exacerbate gut issues, such as certain foods or stressors. This may require keeping a food journal to track symptoms and identify patterns, allowing for targeted elimination of problematic foods.

In practice, an advanced gut healing protocol could involve reintroducing foods in phases following an initial phase of elimination, with an emphasis on nutrient-dense foods that support gut repair; it might also involve adding fermented foods, such as sauerkraut or kimchi, to support a healthy gut microbiome; regular consumption of prebiotic-rich foods, like onions, garlic, and asparagus, can also nourish beneficial gut bacteria; and finally, by combining these dietary strategies with specific lifestyle adjustments, people can improve their gut health and maximize the benefits of their AIP diet for the management of autoimmune conditions.

TAKING CARE OF CO-EXISTING CONDITIONS

While many people with autoimmune disorders also experience symptoms related to other chronic health issues, such as thyroid disorders, adrenal dysfunction, or chronic fatigue syndrome, addressing co-existing conditions in the context of an advanced AIP diet involves identifying and managing additional health challenges that may accompany autoimmune disorders. The comprehensive approach of the AIP diet aims to address these co-existing conditions by promoting overall health, reducing inflammation, and supporting immune function.

Working with healthcare providers who recognize the interdependence of autoimmune diseases and other health conditions is crucial to addressing co-existing conditions effectively. This may entail coordinating care amongst specialists, such as integrative medicine practitioners for holistic management or endocrinologists for thyroid disorders; the AIP diet offers a basis for addressing these conditions through dietary modifications that emphasize foods high in nutrients and eliminate triggers that may exacerbate symptoms.

When it comes to managing co-occurring conditions, a multidisciplinary approach combining targeted medical treatments or therapies with dietary modifications may be necessary.

For instance, people with adrenal fatigue may benefit from dietary modifications combined with stress-reduction techniques like yoga or meditation. Including these strategies in daily life can help manage symptoms effectively and enhance overall quality of life. By adopting a holistic approach to health management, people can navigate the complexities of co-existing conditions while optimizing the benefits of the AIP diet for autoimmune support.

The AIP protocol is not just a short-term diet but a lifestyle approach aimed at managing autoimmune conditions and promoting overall vitality. Long-term maintenance includes cultivating habits that prioritize nutrient-dense foods, stress management, adequate sleep, and regular physical activity—all of which are crucial for maintaining immune function and reducing inflammation. Long-term lifestyle integration in an advanced AIP diet involves adopting sustainable habits that support ongoing health and wellness.

Developing a community of support, whether via online forums or local groups, can also offer encouragement and helpful hints for maintaining the AIP lifestyle over time. If you want to successfully incorporate the AIP diet into your lifestyle, concentrate on creating a supportive environment that encourages healthy choices. This may entail meal planning and preparation to make sure you have AIP-compliant meals easily accessible, even during busy times. It may also involve developing strategies for dining out or social gatherings to navigate food choices while adhering to the AIP guidelines.

The AIP diet is a flexible framework that evolves with your health journey; by viewing it that way, you can cultivate sustainable habits that support long-term wellness and vitality. Embracing these principles into your daily life empowers you to take charge of your health and thrive despite challenges related to your autoimmune condition. In practical terms, long-term maintenance involves periodically reassessing your health goals and making necessary adjustments to your diet and lifestyle. This may include regular check-ins with healthcare providers to monitor progress, update lab tests, and refine your approach to managing autoimmune symptoms.

CHAPTER TEN

HANDLING SOCIAL CIRCUMSTANCES

While adhering to the Autoimmune Protocol (AIP) diet, and navigating social situations can be difficult, it is doable with a few strategies. When you go to social events, it is beneficial to let the host or restaurant knows about your dietary requirements in advance. You should also gently explain the restrictions of the AIP diet and offer to bring a dish that you will enjoy and share with others. This will ensure that you have something to eat and will also inform others about your dietary needs.

At parties, put more emphasis on the company than the food. Talk to people and participate in activities to divert attention from food-focused events. If you can't find many AIP-friendly options, go for basic options like grilled meats, raw veggies, and fresh fruit. Be ready to answer questions regarding your diet; take this as an opportunity to discuss the advantages of the AIP approach to managing autoimmune conditions.

Finally, be kind to yourself. Recognize that not every social gathering will accommodate all of your dietary requirements, and that's alright. Make plans in advance, be upbeat, and keep in mind that following the AIP diet in social situations is worth the effort if it will help you achieve your health goals.

AFFORDABLE AIP RECIPES

Budget-friendly meals on the AIP diet are achievable with careful planning and selection of ingredients. Begin by concentrating on inexpensive staples such as seasonal fruits, root vegetables, and inexpensive cuts of meat or fish. Plan your meals around these ingredients to get the most out of them nutritionally while minimizing expenses.

Preparing big quantities of AIP-compliant meals that can be portioned and frozen for later use is a terrific way to save time and money.

By using materials properly, batch cooking not only minimizes cooking time on busy days but also saves food waste.

Look for fresh food and meats from budget stores and local markets; buying in bulk or during specials can help you save even more money. If you have the space, consider growing your herbs or veggies to add freshness to your meals without spending extra money.

You can make a lot of great AIP meals without breaking the bank if you are creative and resourceful. Try different recipes, adjust for seasonal items, and focus on nutrient-dense foods to help you reach your health objectives while keeping costs down.

ON THE AIP DIET, DINING OUT

When dining out, follow the AIP diet with careful planning and communication. Look up the menu online or give a restaurant a call to find out what alternatives are AIP-friendly; most can accommodate dietary restrictions with advance notice.

When dining out, steer clear of complicated ingredients and stick to basic dishes like plain salads with olive oil and lemon dressing, grilled or steamed meats, and marinades. You can also be wary of hidden ingredients in sauces, dressings, and marinades by asking your server nicely about the ingredients and preparation techniques.

If you can't find anything to eat, try having a small meal before to prevent hunger, or pack a portable, AIP-compliant snack. Being organized lets you enjoy social events without sacrificing your diet.

Finally, thank the restaurant personnel for their efforts to accommodate your dietary needs. Goodwill exchanges can build understanding and motivate businesses to provide more alternatives on their menus for those who follow AIP or other specialized diets.

AIP DIET AND SUPPLEMENTS

While the AIP diet focuses on nutrient-dense whole foods, certain people may benefit from additional supplements to maximize their recovery path. Supplements can complement the AIP diet by addressing particular nutritional needs and promoting overall health.

Important supplements that are frequently suggested on the AIP diet are digestive enzymes to help with nutrient absorption, probiotics for gut health, vitamin D for immune support, and omega-3 fatty acids (from fish oil or algae). These supplements can help fill in nutritional gaps and support the body's healing process.

Before beginning any supplement regimen, it is imperative to speak with a healthcare provider or registered dietitian experienced in the AIP diet. They can evaluate your unique needs, suggest supplements that are appropriate for you, and track your progress to ensure the best possible health outcomes.

As you focus on eating nutrient-dense foods that support your body's recovery, keep in mind that supplements are meant to complement a healthy diet rather than replace it.

You should view supplements as a helpful tool to increase your general well-being when following the AIP diet.

MANAGING MISTAKES AND SETBACKS

The path to better health includes navigating setbacks and blunders on the AIP diet. It's critical to approach these situations with empathy and an emphasis on learning rather than self-criticism. Recognize that setbacks are normal and offer chances for improvement and dietary habit improvement.

If you make a mistake, like eating something that isn't compliant by accident or because of circumstances beyond your control, own it without feeling guilty. Think back on what went wrong and devise ways to avoid it happening again.

Some ideas include organizing your meals more effectively, telling people about your dietary requirements, or using different coping techniques in social situations.

When faced with obstacles, practice resilience and mindfulness. Reduce stress and redirect your attention to your health objectives by engaging in activities like deep breathing, writing, or meditation. Surround yourself with people who are encouraging who understand your journey and can offer support when things become hard.

Remember that every little step you take toward adopting the AIP lifestyle adds to your overall resilience and well-being in treating autoimmune disorders. Keep an optimistic outlook and acknowledge your accomplishments, no matter how minor.